HEPATITIS C

FINALLY ANSWERED ALL THE QUESTIONS

ON HEALING HEPATITIS C

DR. A. RAMOS

Contents

INTRODUCTION

The virus that causes hepatitis C mostly damages the liver by inflaming it and perhaps causing long-term damage. HCV (Hepatitis C virus) is the name of the virus that causes hepatitis C. A thorough explanation of hepatitis C is provided below:

Crucial Points:

Transmission:

Contact with an infected person's blood is the main way that hepatitis C is spread. Common means of transmission include intravenous drug users sharing needles, risky medical procedures, and getting tainted blood or blood products prior to the implementation of broad screening programs.

Prolonged Infection:

Acute and chronic infections can result from hepatitis C. A chronic infection is one that lasts over time, however some people may be able to overcome the virus on their own during the acute phase.

inflammation of the liver:

Inflammation results from the virus's targeting of liver cells. Long-term liver cirrhosis, liver fibrosis, and an elevated risk of liver cancer can result from chronic hepatitis C, even though it might grow silently for years without showing any signs.

Manifestations:

An acute hepatitis C infection may show no symptoms at all or only very mild ones. It's possible that extensive liver damage from chronic hepatitis C won't show any signs at first. Joint discomfort, weariness, jaundice, and stomach ache are possible symptoms.

Hazardous Elements:

Hepatitis C risk factors include sharing personal objects like toothbrushes and razors with an infected individual, having a mother who has the virus, having received blood transfusions or organ transplants prior to widespread screening, and having a history of injectable drug use.

Preventive measures:

Avoiding high-risk behaviors like sharing needles, having safe sexual relations, getting tattoos and piercings done with sterile equipment, and making sure infection control is implemented correctly in hospital settings are all examples of preventative actions.

Assessment:

Blood testing to find HCV antibodies and viral RNA are part of the diagnosis process. Testing liver function is one way to determine the degree of liver damage.

Intervention:

There are antiviral drugs available to treat hepatitis C. The purpose of treatment is to eradicate the virus, lessen inflammation of the liver, and avoid long-term consequences. Treatment plans and lengths can change depending on the individual and the particular HCV genotype.

Progress in Medical Care:

With the introduction of direct-acting antiviral (DAA) drugs, which have fewer side effects and longer half-lives while offering high cure rates for hepatitis C, the therapy for the disease has advanced significantly in recent years.

Impact Worldwide:

Millions of individuals worldwide are impacted by hepatitis C, which is a global health concern. It is a major factor in the morbidity and death caused by liver disease.

Examining and determining:

People who are at risk should get tested for hepatitis C, and screening is an essential part of public health initiatives to detect and treat infections early.

Immunization

Hepatitis C is not currently vaccine-able, in contrast to hepatitis A and B. Reducing the hazards of transmission is the mainstay of prevention.

For the sake of prevention, early detection, and prompt response, it is imperative to comprehend the transmission, dangers, and possible outcomes of hepatitis C. Improved outcomes and a lighter toll from this viral illness are anticipated because to developments in medical research and treatment options. The treatment of hepatitis C mostly involves routine medical exams and adherence to preventive measures.

CHAPTER ONE

Reasons and Hazards

The Hepatitis C virus (HCV) is the primary cause of Hepatitis C, and the main way that it spreads is through coming into touch with an infected person's blood. Preventing and detecting hepatitis C requires an understanding of its causes and risk factors. These are the main reasons and danger signs:

Touching Contaminated Blood:

Direct contact with the blood of an infected individual is the most frequent method of transmission. exchanging needles or other injecting equipment, getting a tattoo or piercing with tainted equipment, or exchanging personal goods like toothbrushes or razors can all lead to this.

Drug Use for Injection:

One of the main ways that intravenous drug users might spread hepatitis C is via sharing needles and other drug paraphernalia. If blood gets on used needles or equipment, it can harbor the virus.

Unsafe Medical Practices:

Before the introduction of broad screening programs, hepatitis C was spread by unsanitary medical procedures such the use of tainted needles and syringes, blood transfusions, and organ transplants.

Healthcare Personnel:

In environments where infection control procedures are not carefully adhered to, healthcare personnel may be at danger if they come into touch with the blood or bodily fluids of infected patients.

Transmission from Mother to Child:

Hepatitis C can be passed from an infected mother to her unborn child during childbirth, although it is less common than hepatitis B. If the mother's viral load is high, the danger is increased.

Dangerous Sexual Behaviors:

Engaging in unsafe sexual behaviors, particularly when other risk factors are present, can contribute to the transmission of hepatitis C, even though the risk of sexual transmission is thought to be lower than that of hepatitis B or HIV.

Transplanting organs and giving blood:

Receiving organ transplants or blood transfusions from infected donors constituted a concern prior to the introduction of standard hepatitis C screening. This risk has been greatly decreased by better screening procedures.

Dialysis of the heart:

Patients receiving long-term hemodialysis may be more vulnerable because of the possibility of coming into contact with polluted shared areas and equipment.

Body piercings and tattoos:

There is a chance of contracting hepatitis C when getting body piercings or tattoos in unsanitary surroundings or with unsterilized equipment.

Many Partners in Sexual Activity:

The chance of coming into contact with contaminated blood or bodily fluids increases when one has several sexual partners, particularly if barrier techniques like condoms are not used.

Coinfection with HIV:

Due to common risk factors and possible mechanisms of transmission, people living with HIV are more likely to get hepatitis C.

The Past of Imprisonment:

People who have served time in prison before are more likely to have hepatitis C, which could be caused by things like drug injection within prisons.

To put preventive measures and focused screening efforts into action, it is imperative to comprehend these causes and risk factors. It is possible to prevent and treat hepatitis C, and early discovery can result in more successful treatment and better outcomes. In order to combat the global burden of hepatitis C, public health programs concentrate on lowering transmission risks and raising awareness.

The symptoms of a hepatitis C infection might differ and it can be acute or chronic. During the early stages of infection, many people with hepatitis C may not exhibit any symptoms at all. Should symptoms manifest, they may be minor or severe. The following are the symptoms and indicators of hepatitis C:

Hepatitis C with an acute case:

Phase without symptoms: People with acute hepatitis C frequently do not show any symptoms at all. When symptoms do arise, they usually show up two to twelve weeks after the virus was first exposed.

Fatigue, fever, and muscular aches are among the flu-like symptoms that some people may encounter.

nausea and loss of appetite: People who have acute hepatitis C may feel sick to their stomachs and lose their appetite.

Pain in the Abdomen: Abdominal pain, particularly in the vicinity of the liver, can happen.

Jaundice: Jaundice can occasionally occur and result in skin and eye discoloration. Pale colored feces and dark urine are also possible.

Pruritus, or itchy skin, is one sign of acute hepatitis C.

Hepatitis C chronic:

For many years, chronic hepatitis C generally advances without causing any discernible symptoms.

Fatigue: People with chronic hepatitis C frequently experience persistent fatigue.

Jaundice: This is a sign of more serious liver damage that some people may experience even during the chronic phase.

Abdominal Pain: Prolonged pain or discomfort in the abdomen, particularly in the area of the liver.

Pale stools and dark urine: During the chronic phase, these symptoms may linger.

Joint Pain: People who have chronic hepatitis C may feel stiffness or pain in their joints.

Cognitive Problems: When hepatitis C reaches an advanced stage, it can impair cognitive function and cause memory and concentration problems.

The majority of people with chronic hepatitis C may not exhibit symptoms until there is substantial liver damage, which is an important point to remember. In order to identify and treat hepatitis C, routine medical exams and screenings are essential, particularly for those who are more vulnerable.

Cirrhosis, or liver scarring, and a higher risk of liver cancer are severe side effects of long-term hepatitis C. Antiviral drugs can effectively prevent or slow down the disease's progression, as well as lower the risk of consequences, with early detection and treatment.

People should seek medical attention for appropriate testing and evaluation if they have concerns about their exposure to or symptoms of hepatitis C. Blood tests to look for viral RNA and HCV antibodies may be part of the testing process. In the event that hepatitis C is discovered, medical professionals can decide on the best course of action, which may involve medication and continuous observation.

Assessment and Diagnosis

In order to confirm the virus's presence, gauge the degree of liver damage, and recommend the best course of treatment, hepatitis C is diagnosed and evaluated using a variety of tests and evaluations. The following are the essential steps in the diagnosis and assessment of hepatitis C:

1. Physical examination and medical history:

In addition to taking a complete medical history that includes hepatitis C risk factors, a healthcare professional will undertake a physical examination to look for symptoms and signs of liver disease.

2. Tests on Blood:

The diagnosis of hepatitis C and evaluation of liver function both depend on blood testing. It is possible to do the following blood tests:

HCV Antibody Test: The existence of antibodies against the hepatitis C virus is detected by this test, which indicates viral exposure. To confirm a current infection, more testing is necessary if the result is positive.

HCV RNA Test: This test determines whether an active infection is present in the blood by identifying the genetic material (RNA) of the hepatitis C virus.

Tests for liver function: These assess the blood's concentrations of various chemicals, including liver enzymes, to determine the health and function of the liver.

HCV Genotype Test: This test determines the hepatitis C virus's particular genotype or strain. Given that distinct genotypes may react differently to antiviral drugs, it aids in guiding treatment decisions.

3. Liver Imaging

To evaluate the structure of the liver and find any indications of cirrhosis or liver disease, imaging tests like MRIs, CT scans, or ultrasounds may be carried out.

4. Liver Elastography or Biopsy:

A liver biopsy could be advised in specific circumstances in order to determine the extent of liver cirrhosis or fibrosis. As an alternative, liver stiffness can be measured using the non-invasive technique of elastography, which serves as an indirect predictor of fibrosis.

5. fibroScan:

Liver stiffness is measured by ultrasonography in the non-invasive FibroScan technique. It gives information on the extent of liver fibrosis.

6. Test for viral loads:

The hepatitis C virus concentration in the blood is determined by the viral load test. It aids in determining the infection's severity and might be used to track how well a treatment is working.

7. Evaluation of Liver Complications and Damage:

Alpha-fetoprotein (AFP) testing for liver cancer and screening for other chronic liver disease consequences are two more tests that may be used to evaluate for liver damage.

CHAPTER TWO

8. Assessment for Hepatitis C-Related Disorders:

Since coexisting disorders might affect treatment options, individuals with hepatitis C may be examined for coexisting conditions such as HIV or hepatitis B.

9. Assessment for Eligibility for Treatment:

The findings of diagnostic tests will be used by healthcare professionals to assess a patient's eligibility and suitability for antiviral therapy. The degree of liver disease, the HCV genotype, and general health may all be taken into consideration when choosing a course of treatment.

To start therapy on time and stop the progression of liver damage associated to hepatitis C, early identification and evaluation are essential. People who exhibit symptoms or are at risk of contracting hepatitis C should consult a doctor so they can get tested and evaluated appropriately. Effective management of the illness requires routine monitoring and follow-ups.

Methods of Treatment

Since the discovery of very powerful antiviral drugs known as direct-acting antivirals (DAAs), the management of hepatitis C has undergone major change. Achieving sustained virologic response (SVR), or the elimination of the virus from the bloodstream following treatment, is the aim of hepatitis C treatment. The mainstays of hepatitis C treatment strategies are as follows:

1. Drugs that fight viruses:

The mainstay of treatment for hepatitis C is the use of direct-acting antivirals, or DAAs. These drugs directly inhibit the hepatitis C virus by targeting particular stages of the virus' lifecycle. When compared to earlier treatments, DAAs have demonstrated significant cure rates for a variety of HCV genotypes and shorter treatment durations.

2. Combination Treatment:

In order to optimize efficacy and reduce the possibility of developing drug resistance, hepatitis C treatment frequently entails combining two or more DAAs. A person's overall health, the degree of liver damage, and their HCV genotype are some of the criteria that determine the exact mix and length of treatment.

3. Customized Therapy Schedules:

Individualized treatment plans are created based on the patient's medical history, HCV genotype, liver disease severity (cirrhosis or fibrosis), and co-occurring diseases. In order to customize treatment plans for every patient, medical professionals thoroughly evaluate these variables.

4. Length of Treatment:

The particular antiviral drugs utilized as well as individual circumstances can affect how long a patient has to get treatment. Nowadays, many regimens are shorter, usually lasting between 8 and 12 weeks, which makes them more patient-friendly.

5. Observation and Prompting:

To evaluate the antiviral therapy's response, routine monitoring is necessary both during and after treatment. Tests for liver function and detecting viral load are part of this. Sustained virologic response (SVR), which denotes a successful virus clearance, is confirmed by post-treatment follow-ups.

6. Transplantation of the liver:

Liver transplantation may be considered in cases where cirrhosis or advanced liver disease have resulted from hepatitis C. Effective antiviral therapies are now more widely available, though, and some recipients may choose to receive antiviral therapy either before to or during transplantation.

7. Modifications to Lifestyle:

For those who have hepatitis C, leading a healthy lifestyle is crucial. This entails abstaining from alcohol, eating a healthy, balanced diet, exercising frequently, and taking care of other risk factors that might affect the health of your liver.

8. Handling of Conditions That Coexist:

To enhance overall health results, healthcare providers may treat coexisting illnesses in addition to hepatitis C treatment, such as HIV or hepatitis B.

Hepatitis C patients must collaborate closely with their medical professionals to create a personalized treatment plan. The field of hepatitis C therapy is constantly changing as a result of continued research into antiviral drugs and other therapeutic modalities.

In addition to eliminating the virus, effective therapy lowers the likelihood of side effects such liver cancer and cirrhosis. Positive outcomes in the management of hepatitis C are largely dependent on early detection, prompt intervention, and adherence to recommended treatment regimens.

Dietary and Lifestyle Factors

Maintaining a healthy lifestyle and choosing food wisely can help manage hepatitis C and improve liver function in general. Although there is no cure for hepatitis C, changing one's lifestyle can improve one's health in spite of the illness. Here are some food and lifestyle suggestions for hepatitis C:

1. Refrain from alcohol:

Alcohol can hasten the onset of liver disease and worsen liver damage. Alcohol drinking is severely discouraged for those who have hepatitis C.

2. Keep a Well-Balanced Diet:

For general health, a diet rich in nutrients and well-balanced is essential. Consume a range of entire grains, fruits, vegetables, lean meats, and healthy fats in your diet.

3. hydration

Maintaining hydration is crucial for liver health. Maintaining a healthy weight and promoting normal liver function are two benefits of drinking enough water.

4. Cut Back on Sugar and Processed Foods:

Processed meals and added sugars may not include necessary nutrients and can add to an excessive calorie intake. It is better for general health to consume fewer processed meals and sugar-filled beverages.

5. Keep Your Weight in Check:

For those with hepatitis C, it's critical to reach and maintain a healthy weight. Being overweight can aggravate fatty liver disease, which can impair liver function.

6. Work Out Frequently:

Frequent exercise supports liver function, among many other health benefits. Physical activity promotes cardiovascular health, helps people maintain a healthy weight, and may even improve general wellbeing.

7. Engage in Safe Sexual Behavior:

Although the risk is thought to be smaller than that of HIV or hepatitis B, hepatitis C can be spread through unprotected sexual contact. The risk of transmission can be decreased by engaging in safe sexual behavior, which includes using barrier techniques like condoms.

8. Refrain from Sharing Personal Items:

It is possible to spread hepatitis C via sharing personal things like toothbrushes and razors that could come into contact with blood. To lower the chance of transmission, don't share these goods.

9. Immunization against Hepatitis A and B:

Hepatitis C patients may be more likely to also have hepatitis A or hepatitis B concurrent infections. To stop further liver problems, vaccination against these viruses is advised.

10. Control your stress:

Long-term stress can affect liver health as well as general health. It may help to practice stress-reduction methods like yoga, meditation, or mindfulness.

11. Consult with Medical Professionals:

It's crucial that people with hepatitis C speak with their medical professionals before making any big dietary or lifestyle adjustments. Based on each patient's unique health requirements and the particular course of hepatitis C, healthcare professionals can provide tailored advice.

In order to create a thorough management plan that include antiviral therapy, routine medical monitoring, and lifestyle modifications, people with hepatitis C must collaborate with their healthcare professionals. For those with hepatitis C, making educated decisions about their food, exercise routine, and general health can help them live longer and better.

Coping Mechanisms and Emotional Health

In addition to medical treatment, managing the psychological and emotional elements of living with a chronic illness such as hepatitis C is essential. The following are some coping mechanisms and pointers for preserving mental health while dealing with hepatitis C:

1. Education and Comprehension:

To improve your knowledge of the virus, how it spreads, and available treatments, educate yourself on hepatitis C. Having knowledge gives people the ability to actively engage in healthcare decision-making.

2. Honest Communication:

Talk to a mental health professional, your family, or supportive friends about your feelings and concerns. Stress can be reduced and a network of support can be established with open communication.

3. Look for Support Organizations:

A sense of camaraderie and shared experiences can be obtained by joining a support group for hepatitis C patients. It can be reassuring and empowering to connect with those going through similar struggles.

4. Assistance for Mental Health:

If you're having emotional problems or obstacles, think about getting help from a mental health expert like a therapist or counselor. They can offer coping mechanisms and resources for handling tension and anxiety.

5. Make sensible goals:

Make sure you set realistic goals for yourself regarding daily activities and treatment adherence. Acknowledge your progress along the route and celebrate tiny successes.

6. Utilize Stress-Reduction Methods:

Take up stress-relieving hobbies like yoga, deep breathing techniques, or mindfulness meditation. These routines have the potential to enhance emotional health and relaxation.

7. Keep Up Your Social Networks:

Maintain relationships with loved ones. Spending time with loved ones can provide one a sense of normalcy and support, which is crucial for mental well-being.

8. Emphasize Self-Care:

Make relaxing and joyful self-care activities a priority. Hobbies, time spent outside, and engaging in activities that encourage a positive outlook are a few examples of this.

9. Take Action Against Stigma:

Acknowledge and dispel any myths or stigma associated with hepatitis C. Advocacy and education are powerful tools for fostering understanding and tearing down barriers.

10. Keep Up With Treatment Information:

Remain updated on the most recent developments in the management of hepatitis C syndrome. Anxiety can be reduced by being aware of the expected results, possible adverse effects, and treatment plan.

11. Adopt a Positive Perspective:

Take proactive measures to maintain your health and cultivate a good outlook by concentrating on your controllable aspects. Thinking positively can enhance general wellbeing.

12. Honor major achievements:

Celebrate and recognize progress made during treatment. Take some time to acknowledge your accomplishments and tenacity, whether it's finishing a course of therapy or accomplishing a personal objective.

13. Consult with Medical Professionals:

Keep lines of communication open with your medical staff. Talk about any emotional or psychological difficulties you may be having, and as part of your overall treatment, work together to address them.

Recall that controlling hepatitis C requires a strong focus on mental health. Even while having a chronic illness might present obstacles, there are ways to maintain a more balanced and fulfilling life, such as finding assistance, taking care of your mental health, and continuing to engage in enjoyable activities.

Liver Function and Problems

Since the hepatitis C virus predominantly targets the liver, causing inflammation and possibly long-term consequences, liver health is an important consideration for those who have the illness. Managing hepatitis C requires understanding liver health, keeping an eye out for problems, and implementing lifestyle changes. An outline is provided here:

1. Hepatic Health:

One of the body's most important organs, the liver is involved in metabolism, detoxification, and protein synthesis. If ignored, a chronic hepatitis C infection can cause hepatitis, or inflammation of the liver, which can worsen liver damage.

2. Stages of Hepatitis:

Hepatitis C can cause liver disease to evolve through many phases, from mild inflammation to advanced cirrhosis and fibrosis (scarring). A late-stage liver disease called cirrhosis is characterized by significant scarring that may compromise liver function.

3. Adverse effects of hepatitis C:

Chronic hepatitis C is frequently accompanied by the following complications:

Cirrhosis: Severe hepatic tissue scarring.

Liver Cancer (Hepatocellular Carcinoma): People who have cirrhosis are more likely to get liver cancer.

Liver failure is a condition in which the liver is unable to carry out its vital tasks due to advanced liver disease.

4. Both cirrhosis and fibrosis:

Frequent evaluation, frequently using elastography, FibroScan, or liver biopsies, aids in determining the severity of liver cirrhosis and fibrosis. The prevention or deceleration of liver disease progression necessitates prompt detection and management.

5. Liver Function Examinations:

Liver health is assessed by routine blood tests, also referred to as liver function tests, which quantify the levels of various chemicals and enzymes in the blood. Increased values could point to injury or inflammation of the liver.

6. Research on Imaging:

The liver can be seen and its structure evaluated using imaging tests including MRIs, CT scans, and ultrasounds. These can aid in spotting indicators of cirrhosis, liver cancer, or liver damage.

7. Screening for HCC, or hepatocellular carcinoma:

People who have cirrhosis have a higher chance of getting HCC, or hepatocellular cancer. To find liver cancer early, it may be advised to do routine screening using imaging studies and alpha-fetoprotein (AFP) testing.

8. Antiviral Medicine:

The hepatitis C virus can be eradicated, liver inflammation can be decreased, and additional liver damage can be avoided with a successful antiviral treatment using direct-acting antivirals

(DAAs). Better results are linked to early therapy initiation.

9. Transplantation of the liver:

Liver transplantation may be an option in cases of severe liver disease or liver failure. Although the necessity for transplants has decreased due to advancements in antiviral therapy, some people may still choose to undergo one.

10. Lifestyle Assessments:

Developing a healthy lifestyle helps promote liver health and lower the chance of problems. This includes giving up alcohol, eating a balanced diet, exercising frequently, and avoiding dangerous behaviors.

11. Shots:

Hepatitis C patients should make sure they receive vaccinations against hepatitis A and hepatitis B in order to avoid developing new liver problems.

Upholding liver health and controlling complications linked to chronic hepatitis C necessitates routine medical checkups, adherence to antiviral medication, and lifestyle changes. Hepatitis C patients should collaborate closely with their medical team to provide individualized treatment and continuous observation.

Public Health and Prevention

In order to lessen the prevalence and effects of the virus, public health activities and the prevention of hepatitis C transmission are essential. Key components of hepatitis C preventive and public health initiatives include the following:

1. Awareness and Education:

Hepatitis C, its mechanisms of transmission, and the need of testing and early detection should be the main topics of public health campaigns. Educational programs aid in debunking misconceptions and lessening the stigma attached to the infection.

2. Examining and Vetting:

To find people with hepatitis C, especially those who are more vulnerable, implement extensive testing and screening programs. Accessible, private, and incorporated into standard medical services are the three main goals of testing.

3. Programs for Harm Reduction:

Promote harm reduction initiatives, especially for drug injectors. There are ways to lower the risk of hepatitis C transmission, including needle exchange programs, sterile injection equipment availability, and injection safety education.

4. Safe Donation of Blood and Organs:

Implement stringent protocols to guarantee the security of organ and blood donations. In order to prevent the spread of infectious diseases during medical procedures, this includes testing donated blood and organs for hepatitis C and other illnesses.

CHAPTER THREE

5. Better Healthcare Procedures:

To stop the spread of infections linked to healthcare, healthcare institutions should encourage and implement infection control practices. This covers using safe injection techniques, properly sterilizing medical equipment, and following general safety procedures.

6. Hepatitis A and B vaccination:

Encourage hepatitis A and B vaccination, particularly in groups where there is a higher risk. Multiple hepatitis virus co-infection can make liver damage worse.

7. Limiting the Transmission of Mother to Child:

To find pregnant women who may have hepatitis C, offer prenatal screening. Take preventive action to lower the possibility of mother-to-child transmission after childbirth.

8. Services for Counseling and Support:

Provide guidance and assistance to people suffering from or at risk of hepatitis C. This covers help with substance abuse, counseling for mental health issues, and help navigating healthcare systems.

9. Personalized Interventions for High-Risk Populations:

Create focused interventions for populations who are more likely to contract hepatitis C, such as drug injectors, men who have sex with other men, and people who are incarcerated. Within these groups, customized approaches can target particular risk factors.

10. Integration of Services:

Incorporate testing, treatment, and prevention of hepatitis C into the current healthcare systems. Comprehensive care requires cooperation between community organizations, public health agencies, and healthcare providers.

11. Treatment Availability:

Provide hepatitis C patients with reasonable and efficient access to antiviral therapies. Increasing treatment accessibility is essential to stopping liver disease from getting worse and lowering its spread.

12. Investigation and Observation:

Encourage continued research to expand on our knowledge of hepatitis C and provide guidance for public health initiatives. Monitoring the prevalence, trends, and demographic patterns of hepatitis C is important for surveillance systems.

13. Worldwide Cooperation:

Encourage international cooperation to combat the effects of hepatitis C on a worldwide scale. A comprehensive global response can be facilitated through the sharing of resources, treatment strategies, and best practices.

Public health efforts can effectively reduce the incidence and impact of hepatitis C by implementing a multifaceted approach that includes education, testing, harm reduction, and treatment. Preventing new infections and enhancing the general health of impacted populations require an all-encompassing approach that is guided by evidence-based practices.

Co-occurring diseases and conditions

The general health of those infected with the virus may be impacted by the coinfections and comorbidities linked to hepatitis C. The following list of frequent comorbidities and coinfections with hepatitis C is provided:

1. Coinfection with HIV:

Those who have hepatitis C frequently also have co-infection with the human immunodeficiency virus (HIV). Both viruses can spread through comparable means, such as sharing needles while using drugs or engaging in unprotected sexual activity. For general health, treating both infections is crucial.

2. Concurrent Hepatitis B:

In areas where both viruses are endemic, coinfection with the hepatitis B virus (HBV) is possible. Liver disease may worsen in those who have both hepatitis B and hepatitis C coinfection. For those who do not have immunity, hepatitis B vaccination is advised.

3. Nonalcoholic Steatohepatitis, or NASH, is a type of fatty liver disease.

Nonalcoholic fatty liver disease (NAFLD) and nonalcoholic steatohepatitis (NASH) can both be made worse by hepatitis C. Increased liver fibrosis and inflammation may be caused by the coexistence of several liver diseases.

4. Diabetes type 2:

There is a correlation between having hepatitis C and a higher chance of type 2 diabetes. It's crucial for people with hepatitis C to keep an eye on and control their blood sugar levels, even though the exact mechanisms underlying the two illnesses are still unclear.

5. Heart Disease:

A higher risk of cardiovascular disease has been linked in some studies to persistent hepatitis C infection. It is imperative that individuals with hepatitis C address cardiovascular risk factors, such as high blood pressure and cholesterol.

6. impairment of the kidneys

Hepatitis C may be linked to chronic kidney disease and renal impairment. To properly manage their health, people with both conditions might need specialized care.

7. Lymphoma-Proliferative Conditions:

There is evidence that certain lymphoproliferative diseases, such as B-cell non-Hodgkin lymphoma, are linked to chronic hepatitis C infection. In order to manage these conditions, regular monitoring and cooperation between healthcare providers are crucial.

8. Arthritis Conditions:

Hepatitis C patients may experience rheumatologic disorders, such as mixed cryoglobulinemia, which can cause symptoms like joint pain. A successful hepatitis C treatment program may reduce rheumatologic symptoms.

9. Substance Abuse Disorders:

Substance use disorders, especially injection drug use, are more common in people with hepatitis C. A vital component of comprehensive care is addressing substance use and granting access to harm reduction initiatives.

10. Mental Health Disorders:

Hepatitis C patients may have higher rates of depression and other mental health issues. The significance of offering psychological support and integrated care is highlighted by the impact of hepatitis C on mental health.

11. Hepatic Cirrhosis and Fibrosis:

Advanced liver fibrosis and cirrhosis are possible outcomes of hepatitis C. Hepatocellular carcinoma, or liver cancer, and portal hypertension are among the complications that people with cirrhosis are more likely to experience.

12. Symptoms that Are Not Hepatic:

Hepatitis C can cause problems outside of the liver, known as extrahepatic complications.

These could include autoimmune phenomena, kidney problems, and skin conditions. To manage these manifestations, close observation and coordination with experts are necessary.

It is imperative that healthcare providers manage patients with hepatitis C while taking these coinfections and comorbidities into account. For people with hepatitis C and related disorders, comprehensive care frequently requires a multidisciplinary team that includes hepatologists, infectious disease specialists, mental health practitioners, and other specialists.

Conclusion

In summary, hepatitis C is a viral infection that mainly affects the liver, causing inflammation and possibly serious damage to the organ. With developments in prevention, treatment, and public health initiatives, considerable strides have been made in the understanding and management of hepatitis C over time. To summarize, these are the main points:

Treatment Advancements: Direct-acting antivirals (DAAs) have transformed the management of hepatitis C, providing patients with longer treatment durations and higher rates of cure. In many cases, these drugs cause sustained virologic response (SVR) because they target particular stages in the virus lifecycle.

Public health initiatives: Especially for high-risk populations, prevention initiatives emphasize testing, education, and harm reduction. In addition to screening and treatment initiatives, vaccination against hepatitis A and B helps lower the virus's prevalence and harmful effects.

The effects of chronic hepatitis C on liver health can range from inflammation to fibrosis, cirrhosis, and, in rare circumstances, hepatocellular carcinoma. To avoid complications, it is essential to conduct routine monitoring, identify problems early, and take action quickly.

HIV and other coinfections, as well as comorbidities like fatty liver disease, diabetes, and cardiovascular disorders, are linked to hepatitis C. In order to enhance overall health outcomes, comprehensive care entails addressing these conditions.

Research and Future Directions: Research on developing vaccines, comprehending the immune response, and hepatitis C elimination tactics is still ongoing. The efficacy of prevention and treatment initiatives is improved by developments in telemedicine, digital health, and international cooperation.

Health Disparities: In an effort to address health disparities, all populations—including disadvantaged and high-risk groups—will have fair access to testing, care, and treatment.

Global initiatives and microelimination are two different approaches to addressing the public health threat posed by hepatitis C. Global initiatives seek to eradicate the virus from particular populations or environments.

Coordinated strategies at the local, regional, and global levels are part of these efforts.

Although there has been a lot of progress, there are still issues to be resolved, such as enhancing testing and treatment accessibility, tackling stigma, and maintaining international efforts for eradication. In order to improve the lives of those afflicted by this viral infection, it is imperative that research, awareness, and cooperative efforts remain ongoing in the fight against hepatitis C.

THE END